The Golden Guide to Weight Management

Rebecca Volpe

Contents

Caution

The information in The Golden Guide to Weight Management is intended as an aid to weight loss and weight maintenance, and is not medical advice. If you suffer from a medical condition you should consult your doctor before starting a weight loss and / or exercise regime. If you start exercising after a period of relative inactivity, you should start slowly and consult your doctor if you experience pain, distress or other symptoms.

Introduction

This is NOT a diet, there are no special formulas, no mixing and matching of foods, no eliminating entire food groups and no forbidden foods. There are no strict recipe plans that include expensive, hard to find ingredients. There is not one single food that you are required to eat over and over again and there are no faddy elements to this guide but there are also no quick fixes. If your aim is to lose weight and keep the weight off then it takes time, time to learn how to eat a balanced diet that is nutritious and healthy. You won't have a healthy body by going on a short-term diet which only delivers short-term results. It's about promoting ongoing health by adopting good habits and this is where the golden guide comes in, a simple way of maintaining dietary health for life.

Over the last few years, collectively, we have lost our common sense when it comes to nutrition and our eating habits. The dieting market has been saturated with too many crazy quick-fix ideas and thus has over complicated losing weight and weight management. Recently we have seen an increase in people being drawn into unsustainable fads and people believing in 'super foods' or their opposite 'bad' foods. Fifty years ago obesity was limited but now many countries are facing an obesity epidemic. The reasons for this can be put down to two main factors; our lifestyles don't include enough physical activity meaning we are not expending enough calories and our diets include too much high calorie and high fat foods that we are consuming too frequently.

The answer to combat this growing problem is relatively simple. We have to inform ourselves of what we are consuming and return to a simpler way of eating which consists of fresh natural foods. This simpler, 'cleaner' way not only does the world of good for our bodies but our minds and purses too. Over the past few decades we have seen a sharp increase in the amount being spent on dieting and the many products on offer to those looking for ways to feel good, lose weight and get in shape. However, not only is it our hard earned cash that we are spending too much of we have been spending too much time and energy concerned with slimming, faddy foods, dieting and quick-fix exercise fads. What we should concern ourselves with is healthy eating in a natural way, the rest, losing weight and looking better, will quickly follow.

In this guide you will learn the key elements to gaining and maintaining a healthy balanced way of eating. We look into the psychology of our eating habits and how to be in control of our diet. We also go into the importance of exercise because even if diet is the foundation to losing weight and leading a healthy lifestyle, exercise is the essential element that makes it all work. The good news is that this guide will not make you suffer and it has no adverse side effects like so many fad diets (cabbage soup diet anyone?) in-fact you will gain more energy and feel better in a multitude of ways. You may find that due to your existing diet you suffer from a few unpleasant symptoms like constipation, diarrhoea, headaches, stomach pains, bloating, lethargy, mood swings, irritability, depression and many others, these will ease and more than likely disappear completely when following the guide.

What you put into your body has a huge effect on what you get out of it, I don't know anyone that can honestly say they feel amazing on a diet of fast food and nutrient zapped foods. This guide will teach you how to make healthy choices in your diet so that your body benefits.

It is also a very simple guide, nothing complicated or mathematical, it is purely information and techniques to steer you to a balanced and healthy new you. It is important that you make gradual changes to your diet, don't change everything in one week as it will be too much of a shock for your body if your current diet and exercise regime is less then desirable. I recommend applying one golden point each week and no more. It may seem tempting to 'start fresh' and overhaul your existing diet by following all 15 points at once but changes take time to make and get used to. Plus, if you were to implement just one point each week you can really focus on each point and by the time 15 weeks has passed you will have a much healthier diet that has gradually been adopted- meaning that it will be easier to maintain.

The reason that so many popular diets don't work long-term is that they are unsustainable (how long can you realistically eat only protein for?) leading to ill health and a quick drop in weight but a sudden weight gain shortly after finishing the diet, then repeating this vicious cycle with increased extremes. This constant yo-yo dieting sends the body into panic as it gets sent signs of starvation when it receives well below the necessary amount of calories needed. This in turn will encourage the body to compensate and switch on all the mechanisms it has to store food, especially when the diet has concluded and normal eating is resumed. In-fact nearly 65 percent of dieters return to their pre-dieting weight within three years, according to Gary Foster,

Ph.D., clinical director of the Weight and Eating Disorders Program at the University of Pennsylvania. It gets worse for dieters who lose weight rapidly with only 5 percent of people who lose weight on a crash diet keeping the weight off. This is according to Wellsphere, a website sponsored by Stanford University. Plus, not only is yo-yo dieting physically bad for your body and for maintaining a healthy weight, it also has a negative effect on mindset as a strict deprivation of certain foods and food groups will quickly have you craving it more thus disturbing the balance and will lead to over-eating once the diet is completed. A true recipe for disaster!

This guide contains all the information necessary to change your diet and give your body all that it needs and wants so that it is able to do what you require of it. There is also a bit of space for your very favourite treats, because after all, this is not something you will do for the next six months or until you get to your goal weight and then revert back to old ways, this is a guide for life.

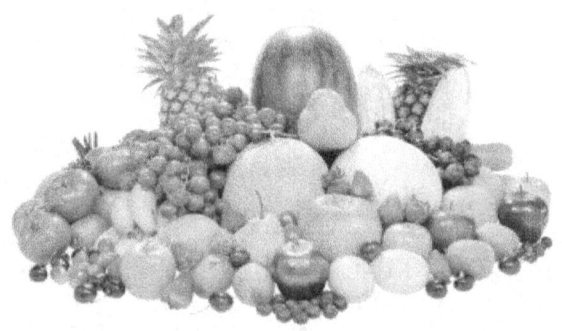

1. Keep a food and exercise diary

Often we go through life in such a rush that we barely notice what we are putting in our bodies and how we are treating them. In order to understand where we are going wrong (and where we are going right) with our diets and exercise regime we must first see what we have been doing. The simplest and most effective way to do this is by keeping a food and exercise diary. By writing down what you eat and drink and what exercise you do it is easier to see where it can be improved. This can be done on a piece of paper or on a mobile phone if you find it more convenient, just as long as you can keep the list with you at all times.

Write down everything that you eat and drink throughout the day and any exercise you have done and most importantly, be honest. It doesn't matter where you write this down but it is important that at the end of the day you can take two minutes to look at it and see where you can improve, what changes you can make and also where you are doing the right things. Visualise what you ate throughout the day and be honest with yourself. Was it too much? Was it healthy? Could it have been better? You can even imagine taking a photo of everything you ate during each day and imagine posting that photo on a social website. Would the photo make you proud of your diet or would you be embarrassed by what you have consumed? You are likely to find that this will help prevent you from over-eating and making bad choices in your diet because you have to write everything down and see it later, you are more likely to go for healthier and better options.

The ideal way to keep a diary is to take a note book or an A4 piece of paper and write down the date at the top. Draw a grid with vertical columns representing each of the following categories; vegetable and fruit, protein, carbohydrates, drinks and finally, treats. For each meal, or every time you eat, fill in the columns horizontally, starting with the time on the left side, by doing this you can see at what times you are eating and understand if this is something that could be changed and improved. For example, maybe you can space out meal times better to avoid feeling hungry late afternoon or you can avoid having a late night snack.

The idea of the grid is that you can fill the vegetable and fruit column as much as you like (well... minimum 5 portions, maximum 8). The third column must contain good sources of protein and calcium like fish, lean meat, eggs, and milk every time you have a meal (at least three times a day but no more than four). The fourth column must have three to five portions (three portions is good if you are watching your weight) of good sources of carbohydrates like sweet potato, brown rice, brown pasta and whole-grain bread. The drinks column should contain at least 8 glasses of water and the treats column should contain as little as possible! Consult the good food list for more ideas of foods that are good to include in your diet.

By knowing that you should be hitting these targets everyday for the things that you do eat it also means that you are more likely to fill-up on the good stuff and leave less room for treats. Plus, by looking at it from a psychological aspect, when you concentrate on the foods that you should eat it moves the focus from foods that you should avoid, making this guide more about the positive aspect of healthy eating than looking at dieting in a negative restricting way. I advise completing a food and exercise diary as one of the first things to do if you want to lose weight or if you are feeling that your are losing control of your diet and exercise regime. Don't think that you need to write down everything you eat for the rest of your life, it's more of a realisation technique for when your eating habits get a little out of control that can be followed through until you gain control or lose the amount of weight you want. By completing the simple task of jotting down what you consume it is much easier to see how you can change for the better. Without writing it down it could be that you may have forgotten you had that doughnut earlier in the day and would have eaten the brownie in the evening too but because it all gets written down you will be more aware of what you have eaten and what you should be eating. Just be honest!

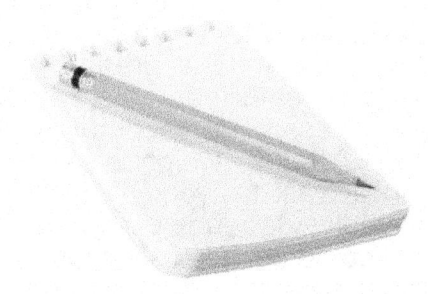

It is also important to write down what exercise you do each day so that you can see if it is enough. Again, being completely honest, write done the type of exercise you did and for how long. I would also advise scoring your day from 1-10 on how active you have been, excluding "official exercise" like gym or a fitness class. Think about extra movement you did, for example, walking up and down the stairs, riding a bike to work, rushing around doing chores. A score of one would be an extremely low level of activity and ten would be a score for a very high amount of activity. Try to aim for the highest number possible by including as much activity as possible in your lifestyle and aim for at least 3 hours of planned exercise each week.

It is a good idea to consult a fitness professional so that they can design a personal fitness program tailored to your specific needs and give advice on performing exercises safely and correctly. Alternatively, find a class or activity that you enjoy so much it doesn't even feel like 'proper exercise', join a dance or fitness class, organise a football game, take up swimming. There are so many great ways to get active that can be fun, social and escapist, you just have to try them out and find the right activity, or two, for you. Another great way of reaching a higher level of general activity in your day is to aim for a certain amount of steps. The recommended amount of steps each day is 10,000, which may seem a lot but when factoring in a walk to work or taking the dog out, this can be achievable. Depending on whether on not you find it helpful, you could consciously measure the amount of steps you take throughout the day with a pedometer, or if you have the discipline, you can make a conscious choice to walk more. It is this type of 'extra activity' that can bring big changes to your lifestyle and thus make you healthier, enable you to lose or maintain weight and generally make for a much more active and happier you.

2. Vary what you eat

There are so many different healthy foods and drinks out there that there is no need to eat the same things over and over again, day in day out. It is important to try different foods, things you may never have tried before and foods that you wrote-off as being disgusting when you were ten years old! Your preferred tastes change over time and so start afresh with an open mind and try a little bit of everything. I knew someone that at the age of twenty-seven had never tried pineapple before because he thought he wouldn't like it, he tried it and loves the fruit now. Nearly everyone has some type of food that they have dismissed long-ago and haven't touched in years, it could be that if you tried it again you might just end up loving it. Sometimes psychological factors and links have put you off eating certain foods in the past but clear that away and try everything, you may be surprised to find a new love of olives or broccoli.

In order to prevent getting bored with your new health plan, vary what you eat as much as possible. Go to the supermarket and take time to have a good look at all the different healthy foods that are available. Pick-up some fruits that you have never tried before, sample different fish or make a simple change from white to brown rice. Also, don't dismiss foods that you consider to only be for 'health nuts' or vegetarians, you may never have tried cous cous or tofu before but how do you know that you don't like it until you have tried it, it could even become a new favourite. Check out the good food list for ideas and try something new.

Not only is it important to vary what you eat for the sake of keeping things interesting and appealing, it's also vital for health reasons and to give your body as many nutrients as possible. Our bodies are complex systems that require certain amounts of many different vitamins and nutrients everyday. Without resorting to taking several different expensive supplements and multi-vitamins, it is possible to get close to the recommended daily amounts through a varied, nutritious diet. The aim should be to pack your diet with super healthy foods and in the biggest range possible; include lot's of different vegetables and fruits, get plenty of variety with your protein and carbohydrate choices and include good quality essential fats. This may seem like a lot to pack in when you are trying to lose or control weight but by being smart about it and including lots of different ingredients, while still controlling the overall portion size, you will be giving your body all that it needs.

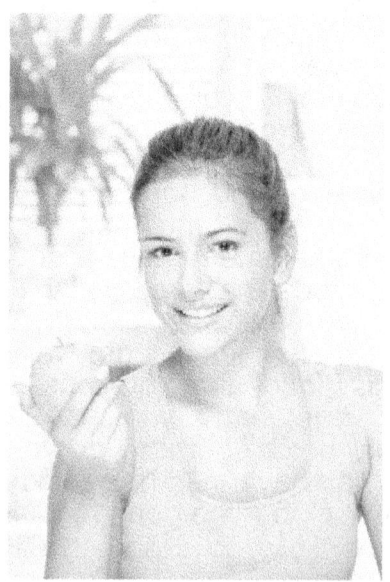

3. Experiment with cooking and preparing food

You may not be winning any cooking competitions or be a five star chef but the good news is you don't have to be in order to improve your diet. When I was at college I would literally have five minutes to prepare my lunch in the morning, I didn't want to have to cook anything so I would make the biggest and best salad you have ever seen. It had everything in it and looked so good my friends would want my lunch rather than their burger and chips. It was the easiest, cheapest and fastest lunch I could do. I would go to the shops at the weekend and buy a bag of ready-cut salad, peppers, cucumber, tomatoes, ham, cheese, tuna, beetroot, radishes, a pot of ready made cous cous, celery, carrots and anything else that I could put in a salad. The morning or night before, I would chop a few things up and throw it all in a plastic box ready to go. It tasted great, it never got boring because I would always vary what I put in the salad, it cost a maximum of ten pounds for a weeks worth of substantial lunches and it was super healthy.

It's not just salads that are easy and fast to do, try making big sandwiches with healthy bread, pasta with a tasty tomato sauce, make up some good quality noodles or a jacket potato with a tasty topping and lots more. Try a little cooking too, it doesn't have to be complicated or celebrity chef worthy but the best way of knowing exactly what you are eating and to be sure that you are getting healthy meals that are free from extra sugars, additives and salts, is to prepare it yourself. So often people who want to lose weight are choosing 'saintly' options from the local cafe or shop unaware of exactly what is inside and all the 'extras' that add up to a calorie loaded bomb!

For example, a simple chicken salad may contain nearly as mainly calories and grams of fat as a full roast dinner due to the added dressing or croutons. If you were to make a similar meal at home you can control what you are putting into it and how it is made and therefore exactly what you are eating. Plus it will be so much cheaper than buying ready-made from the shops each day. Check ideas on the internet for simple recipes that are tasty and good for you. Everyone can manage to grill fish and boil some rice and vegetables so don't be worried and give it a go.

The other advantage of cooking meals yourself is that you can adjust the methods of cooking to maintain as much of the original nutrition from the ingredients as possible. Steaming vegetables is the best method to retain as much of their vitamins and minerals as possible. Also, unlike frying or roasting, oil is not needed and not absorbed by the vegetables therefore eliminating extra calories and fat. Grilling and poaching are also healthy options for home cooking and just this little alteration can make a big difference.

That's not to say that you can't eat-out or get a takeaway ever again but it's best to look at it as more of a treat, an option that can be part of a healthy lifestyle but balanced out with the majority of your meals being healthy and homemade. Basically, whatever your situation is, there is always a way to eat something good. Experiment in your kitchen a little and you will find that the food you make will be healthier and more rewarding than buying a takeaway.

4. Make healthier choices

Little tweaks to your diet are often the best way to make it healthier and it doesn't take much to make a big difference. By finding alternatives to high calorie and high fat foods and drinks that still satisfy your taste-buds you can make a big overall difference. For example, if a life without ice cream is unthinkable then try looking for alternatives that don't blow your whole day's worth of calories in one sitting, find an alternative that still tastes great but is better for you, chances are you won't even tell the difference.

We are lucky that we have so much choice in the shops so take a little time to go around and find similar but better products. Be careful to pay attention to what is written on the packaging as it may not be as good as what it implys. Lots of "healthy" foods can be full of additives, hidden sugars and fats, so take a good look at the ingredients and nutritional information. Don't fall for the low-fat foods or zero per cent fat products as these products won't be helpful for people wanting to lose weight. When fat is removed, something needs to be added to retain taste and texture, this is usually sugar and flour, which provide calories but are nutritionally poor. A small amount of fat is essential for all of us and it is also very satiating, so a small amount will keep us feeling more satisfied and invariably lead to eating less. Many low-fat products don't satisfy and leave us feeling hungry which leads to eating more and many studies back this up showing that the dieters who lose weight and keep it off eat moderate amounts of fat.

The type of fat consumed is important as there is a big difference between good and bad fats. Aim to consume a small amount of good fats in every meal, such as omega-3 fatty acids which are found in oily fish, walnuts, flax seeds and other sources. Other good fat options are avocados, olive oil, semi-skimmed milk and natural yogurt, foods that naturally contain an amount of fat but are doing you good, unlike the fat from a chocolate cake! Saturated fats found in many cakes, biscuits and other products will not contain any nutritional benefit for the eater in any way and should be kept to a minimum. So if in doubt about your fats, choose 'natural' products as the less they are altered the better and therefore the healthier they will be.

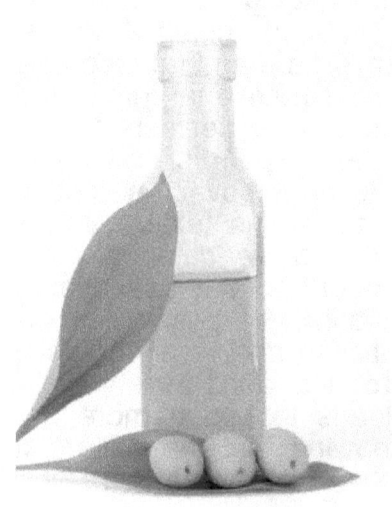

Things like biscuits can easily contain as many as 100 calories each so by changing a chocolate-covered, caramel biscuit to a much more natural and healthier option of oat, fruit and honey biscuit you can make a change for the better. Another area that is easy to make some simple changes to is condiments and sauces. Pay attention to these as many can be very calorie dense which means that by cutting back, or cutting them out completely, you will lower your overall calorie intake and provide an easy way of losing weight.

As a very general rule most sauces that have a white colour will have either a high cream, cheese or egg base to the recipe and will therefore be very high in calories. Try using alternatives to flavour your food and cook with. Extra virgin olive oil, garlic, lemon, herbs and spices are all perfect for seasoning and cooking with. They will add delicious flavour and are also good for you.

Even basic staple foods and drinks can be upgraded to a healthier choice. If you use semi-skimmed milk instead of full-fat you are already eliminating a couple of hundred calories a week. Imagine if you were to trade in all of your regular food and drink choices for the lighter and healthier options. Calories would be kicked away and so would extra weight, all from just a few small tweaks.

5. Every food you eat should contain something nutritious about it

Aim for a diet full of natural, nutritional foods and try eliminating colourings, added flavouring, additives and preservatives. Just by eliminating the bad stuff you will almost certainly be on the way to completing this principle. The aim here is to consume the most nutritional diet you can which will result in good health and losing excess weight. The less processes and changes that your food has gone through the better. Not so long ago we didn't have anything added to our foods, we had to eat fresh food that was locally grown and came without chemical alterations. Now the majority of products that you find in the supermarket will have gone through some kind of alteration process and it's not benefitting us. As humans we were never meant to consume foods that contain all the nasty things that they do today.

If you have a look at the ingredients list on the food packet and can't even pronounce some of them- do you really want to be putting them in your body? Sugar is a key ingredient in many products and really if it appears amongst the first few ingredients the best place for it is back on the shelf. However, it can be listed in various different ways on a label making it trickier to decipher. Code names for sugar can be: corn syrup, maltose, dextrose, sucrose, fructose and anything else ending in 'ose'.

If there is a certain food that you love but fear that it is made in a less than natural way find out how it is made and what exactly is in it. I think it is only right that we truly understand what we are putting into our bodies and having the knowledge of how these foods are made and what they contain may make you think about whether you really want to continue eating it. After seeing how jelly sweets are made I vowed never to eat one again. That's real food for thought!

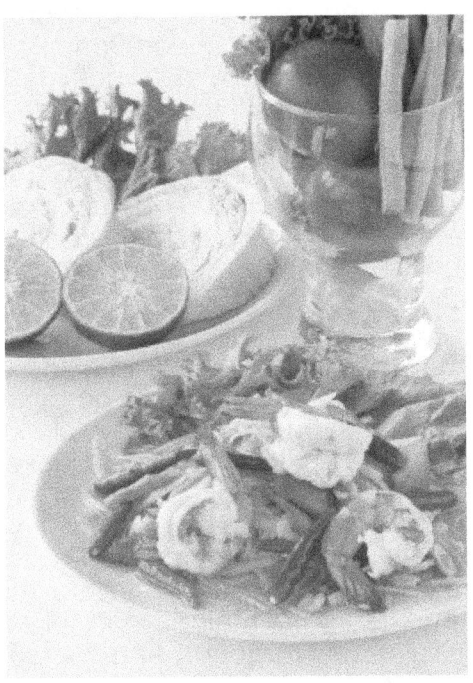

There are a lot of foods out there that are true junk foods which contain no trace of nutritional goodness. The only thing to gain from these foods are fats and probably the worst type of fats at that. Try hard to avoid these by considering before consuming if its really worth eating all those 'empty calories' (food that contains no nutritional value). This doesn't cut out as many 'naughty' foods as you may think. It doesn't mean a life without your favourite treats because even something like chocolate can contain some nutritional value if you choose the right kind. Dark chocolate that contains a large percentage of cocoa (around 80%) has been proven to have some rewarding benefits when eaten in moderation. Even pizza of the healthier kind contains carbohydrates from the bread base, protein from the cheese and if you pile lots of vegetables on top you are also getting vitamins and minerals. However, I stress that it doesn't mean that all pizza is nutritional, a huge stuffed-crust, meat-feast with extra cheese thats swimming in grease and dipped in high-fat mayonnaise is for sure doing more harm than good. As mentioned before, try and choose the healthy options for the food that you eat and avoid any food that doesn't benefit your body in any way.

Another good way to balance your intake of good healthy food verses treats that you love is to go by the 80/20 rule, 80% of the food that you consume in the week is healthy, nutritious food, naturally low in fat and packed full of good nutrients that your body needs to function at its best. The other 20% is for you to enjoy a little of your favourite treats, healthy or not. Many people have adopted this rule and apply it to a weekly format so that during the week a healthy diet is maintained and for one day of the weekend the rules are forgotten and the 20% is enjoyed in the form of a 'treat' day. This can work, but it can still feel depriving and is unsustainable for a long period of time, it's extremely limiting and not a very appealing way to live. It can also result in just looking forward to that one day over the course of the week and ending with a massive blowout, not a very balanced way of eating. All this, plus let's not forget the challenge for your digestive system when it gets shocked by a massive fat-fest!

Healthy eating should make you feel better and not be a penance. The aim is for healthy eating to be just as enjoyable, if not more so, than your previous diet. I would suggest balancing out the treats a little, you could opt to eat healthy in all your meals but enjoy a small treat of a few squares of chocolate, a small glass of wine or something similar each day. This way you won't feel that you are being deprived of the things that you love and crave.

It is always a good idea to include treats in your diet so that you don't build up a feeling of complete depravation that ends in a rummage of the cupboards at midnight, searching for biscuits when you reach breaking point! Even if your very favourite food or drink is nutritionally at the bottom of the healthy list and you would be better off without it you can still include this as your treat, in moderation, because the more you think that it is forbidden, the more your brain will go into overload craving it! It is still possible to lose weight, even when consuming a treat each day as long as there is balance, you are exercising and the treat doesn't push your calorie intake too much (up to 200 calories), then a small treat is fine as part of a balanced diet. Just make sure that you stick to the 80/20 proportions and don't go crazy by eating two weeks worth of calories in one meal when it comes to your treat time!

6. Drink water

Everyone says to do it but few actually do it enough. The benefits of water are endless and it is an imperative part of a healthy diet. The body requires water in countless ways and it is vital you take on enough fluid for your body to function properly. If you feel thirsty it's too late, you are already beginning to be dehydrated. Another sign of dehydration is if you suffer from headaches, top up your water intake and this problem could be solved. The average person should be drinking eight cups of water a day, or roughly two litres. Your requirement will increase when exercising or in hot climates especially if you sweat a lot. However, if you eat plenty of foods that contain a high water content like soups and fruits, you may find that this helps you achieve your target water intake. One simple way of knowing if your getting enough fluid is to check your urine, it should be a very light yellow colour.

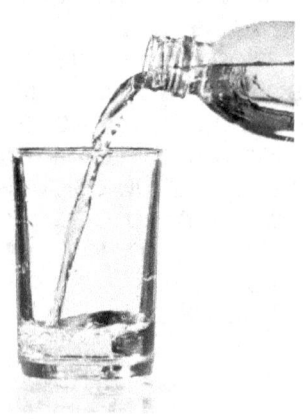

Many people find water boring or tasteless and won't be able to drink the recommended amount of plain water. If this is the case, try adding lemon for flavour or drink flavoured water. Experiment with hot water and lemon too. Water with a bit of juice still counts but make sure its not full of sugar and is mostly water. Tea also counts, the best kinds are flavoured teas, especially green tea for a fat-busting antioxidant boost, but also English tea with a splash of milk will count (just don't add heaps off sugar, try it without or slowly cutting down). Remember, it isn't only drinks that count to your eight glasses a day, eating foods high in water content will boost your hydration, salads, fruits and soups are amongst the foods that contain lots of water, so fill up on these too. Aim to space out getting your two litres by having a big glass of water with every meal and carrying a bottle of water with you to sip from. Dehydration can be confused with the signs of hunger so it's important to stop and think if you could just be in need of water instead of something to eat. Try having at least a couple of sips of water before a meal, by doing this it will help to stop you over-eating if your body is a little dehydrated.

7. Beware the drinks you drink

It often happens that when we think about eating healthily that is exactly what we do, eat healthily and forget about drinking healthily too. Drinking water is super important but it is also important to avoid the drinks that are loaded with empty calories (no nutritional value) and full of sugar or sweeteners. Fizzy drinks are a culprit here, with some containing enough sugar and fat to be the calorie equivalent of a small meal.

Another trap many people fall into is thinking that because it has diet written on the side of the bottle that it is good for you but the majority of these drinks are full of sweeteners, additives and caffeine. Artificial sweeteners can be 13,000 times sweeter than sugar and when the body is hit with this high dose of sweet flavour but doesn't get the calories it expects, sweet cravings will go into over-drive. This upsets the balance, making it extremely hard to avoid sugary foods. Studies have found that people who drink diet-drinks are more likely to be fatter than those that don't. In another study that followed diet-drink consumers over a ten year period it was found that their waists actual grew an amazing 70 per cent more than those that didn't consume diet-drinks.

Not only can diet drinks make it harder for you to control your weight they could also increase the risk of developing type-2 diabetes by 67 per cent. It may take time for a fizzy drink addiction of six-a-day to be brought down to size but slowly, week by week, try to cut down and maybe cut out completely (unless you fancy this as your treat maybe twice a week).

The same goes for alcohol, I am not saying that for the rest of your life you can't touch another drink and you must stay free from alcohol but keep in mind that most alcoholic drinks contain a minimum of 100 calories and some cream-laden cocktails can easily be the equivalent of a Sunday roast! If a drink or two is your chosen treat, you can still enjoy it by balancing out what you eat and putting in an hour of added exercise. Try to find ways of enjoying your drink treats but not in an excessive kind of way. Alternate with water and fruit juice and choose fruit based cocktails and spritzers over creamy calorific ones.

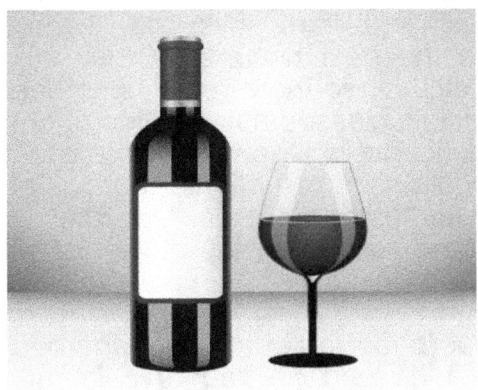

Alcohol and fizzy drinks are responsible for many people's excess weight problems as we are so often unaware of just how many calories and how much fat is contained in the drinks. If you feel that the quality of your fluid intake could be improved, I would suggest trying to consume just water based drinks (ideally just water) with fresh lime or lemon for a brief period. After just a week you will notice the difference to how you feel and probably what you weigh. Another incentive is that you are likely to notice a decrease in bloating and may also be aware that the area around your belly is flatter.

Alcoholic and fizzy drinks are often responsible for bloating due to the high level of sugar content, so if that's not an incentive to cut down, I don't know what is!

Basically try to include as much water as possible in whatever ways possible. A glass of pure fruit juice is a good choice if you struggle to eat your five portions of fruit and veg each day but just remember that because many more portions of fruit go into each pure fruit juice drink, the total amount of calories and natural sugars will be high. This is fine if you're consuming a small glass but not great if your drinking a carton or two each day! Don't forget the all important milk too, semi-skimmed or skimmed are the best options as they still give you a good hit of calcium, so there really is no need to go near the full-fat. Milk is classed as a portion of protein/dairy so it's a great option to include this for breakfast. If you love your hot chocolates look for lighter options or try Ovaltine and malt drinks instead. Herbal teas are a good choice with green tea being at the top of the list with its saintly credentials.

Green tea has been found to assist the body in flushing out excess fluids and helping to calm bloating in the stomach caused by water retention. It has also been found to speed up the metabolism which can aid the burning of excess fat in the body. Now the only thing is that this won't really be effective with just one cup of green tea, several cups a day are needed to get all of the benefits. A simple trick would be to make a small jug (around 1 litre) of boiling water and use several green tea bags (around 5-6) to get a blast of green tea benefits. Once cooled slightly, you could place the tea inside a large shaker or drinks container to carry around with you and drink from over the next hours. A fantastic pre-exercise boost too.

8. Priorities eating and exercise

Don't let eating and exercise be at the very end of your to do list, this is about your well-being and how you feel, it should be at the top of the list. With so many aspects of modern day life, battling it out for a little bit of precious time, it is easy to have meal and exercise time pushed aside. The good news is that with a bit of thought and planning you can easily fit healthy meals and exercise into your day.

Think about ways that you can be more active throughout your normal day; banning the lift and taking the stairs instead, cycling or walking to work, playing a physical game with children or walking the dog. You don't have to be in the gym to be active and get the benefits. Six out of seven days you should try and get active in some way, for example, plan 'proper exercise' for these 6 days, it could be going to the gym, swimming, an exercise class, a football game etc and try hard to stick to it. For the days when life gets in the way and you just can't do your planned exercise make an effort to be more active during the day, take a longer route when walking the dog or if you are shopping, carry the bags around with you instead of dropping them off in the car. Be inventive so that you are generally being more active even if your plan doesn't always go to plan!

The same goes for meals, make a list of foods you need before hitting the supermarket (remember don't pick up unhealthy treats and they won't be tempting you at home) and have an idea of meals you can put together for the week. Check out the 'perfect multi-meal ingredient list' at the end of this guide for a variety of straight forward meals. You may find shopping online for your groceries

29

an advantage as you can take time to check your list without making unnecessary impulse buys and it also means you don't need to be going around the shops when you are hungry. Studies have shown that we are much more likely to pick and purchase products that are high in fat and sugar when we are hungry, so don't fall into that nasty little trap! Also have plenty of 'plan B' meals for the times when you don't have time to cook or, in a really bad case, you don't have time to even stop.

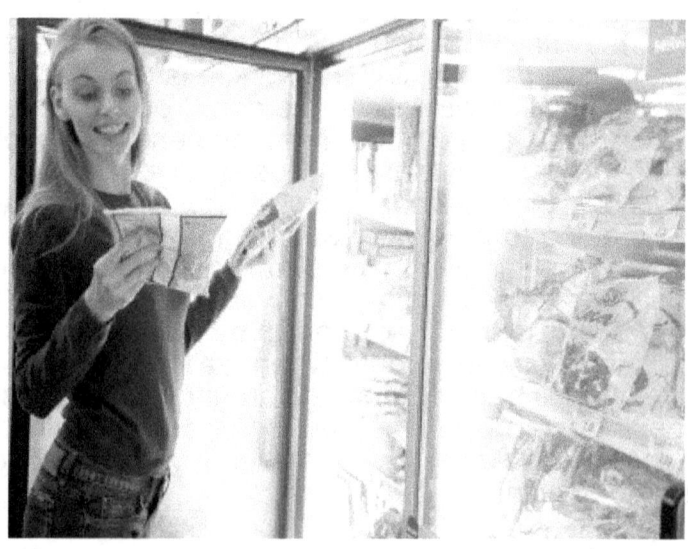

Stock up on items that can be made super fast but don't touch the ready meals. A 'healthy' ready meal may seem like the perfect choice but they are loaded with additives, salt, saturated fat and lots more rubbish, even the 'healthy' ones, so step away. Instead opt for fast cooking pasta or noodles, tins of vegetables, baked beans or whole-wheat toast and scrambled eggs in the microwave- which take less time to prepare than a ready meal. There are plenty of good options even if you only have five minutes to prepare a meal. Of course a great back-up would be to have your own homemade meals frozen and ready to defrost when needed. By making extra portions when you are cooking a regular meal you will have plenty of delicious options waiting for you in the freezer when you have no time to cook.

If you really can't stop, have some healthy snacks ready in the cupboard or in your bag that you can grab. They will keep you going so that you aren't famished when it comes to your next meal and your can avoid blood sugar levels from dropping too low. Stock up on fresh fruit (it is about the easiest and fastest snack), dried fruit, carrot sticks, nuts and seeds as they are all great for quick snacks and can be kept in your bag or at a desk just incase. Low-fat crackers and rice cakes are great choices but always check the labels for hidden nasties. Snacks like cereal bars may seem like an ideal on-the-run snack but they are full of hidden sugars. It is very difficult to find any that are truly healthy so an alternative idea would be to buy the ingredients and make your own. All in all, plan your exercise and meals but always have options in case your best intentions don't always work out.

9. Don't rush eating

If you enjoy eating (and who doesn't?) then why rush the pleasure? Obviously, sometimes life gets in the way and taking time out to enjoy your lunch may seem like a luxury you just don't have but enjoying your meal, making it last and making time to eat in your day can make a real difference. Even think of it as something to look forward to by making it a priority to sit down, relax and forget all the things you have to do and concentrate on the food, taste, texture and everything about the experience of eating good nutritious food.

Try to avoid eating on-the-go or when stood-up, and make it a rule to only eat when sat down. You will instantly eat less by avoiding picking and snacking at unnecessary food. Prioritise eating at a table as it breaks the link of being sat on the sofa and eating, a habit that easily leads to over-eating. When we are distracted by other elements or activities we can be unaware of what and how much we are mindlessly eating.

It takes 20 minutes for signals from your full tummy to reach your brain, so if you have eaten your meal within 15 minutes you will continue eating more than your body requires. Try checking the clock when you take your first mouth-full and again on your last, any less than 20 minutes for a full meal means your rushing and quite possibly over eating. When you eat slower, you will feel fuller on less food than if you gulp it down. This is one of the easiest ways to lose weight- by slowing down and listening to your body.

It may seem strange to eat so slowly if you have been used to fast-paced eating but taking a little time to chew food properly, sip on water in between bites and to enjoy conversation over your meal will help you listen to signals that you are full. This habit will also prevent bloating and improve digestion as eating slowly, while sitting down gives your body a chance to process the food properly.

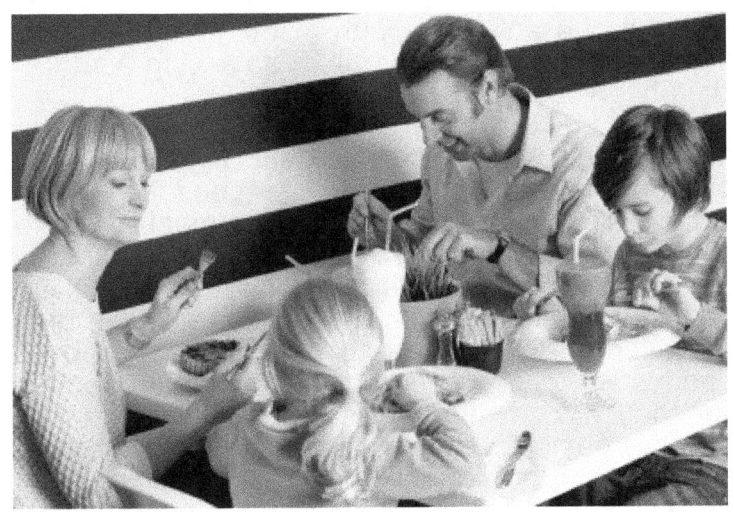

10. Don't wait to be hungry, you don't need to starve yourself and NEVER skip meals.

With this guide you should never feel hungry. When it gets closer to your next meal it is normal to feel more of an appetite building but never really hungry. Use your food diary to understand when you start to get hungry and are in danger of reaching for a chocolate snack. Be prepared for this and have a healthy snack ready, or next time, slightly increase the size of your pre-slump meal. You should be eating enough at meal times to feel full and satisfied but not overly full, a balancing act that with a little observation can be achieved.

Skipping meals, especially breakfast will lead to a drop in blood sugar levels and make you feel hungrier during the day, it causes over-eating at your next meal time or over-eating of unhealthy snacks. You are more likely to crave high-fat and sugary foods as you are craving calorie dense food, making it painfully hard to resist the biscuits. Binge eating is more likely to happen at night because the body tries to catch-up on missed calories from earlier in the day. Blood sugar levels need to be maintained during the day and the best way to do this is to eat at regular times throughout the day, including snacks. Generally, as the day goes on we are in need of less and less calories until we wind down and go to bed therefore it makes sense that the highest percentage of daily calories is consumed in the first half of the day.

Having a substantial breakfast, a good lunch and a smaller dinner that is punctuated with healthy snacking, is the optimum distribution of calories and therefore energy. Many of us have been brought-up, or have to work around, a small or almost non-existent breakfast and lunch followed by a king sized dinner that will sit in the stomach until bed time. It may take a while to flip this habit but once you succeed you will certainly feel better for it because the balance evens out energy levels providing you with a boost when you need it most.

Breakfast is especially important because the body has gone without food throughout the night and requires nutritious food to pick-up the blood sugar levels and get the body going but also to be able to provide enough energy to function well throughout the morning. So break-the-fast and have breakfast! Even if you can't manage to face a full meal in the morning just a small amount of something nutritious will go a long way in preventing those cravings later on. Try a yoghurt and fruit, a slice of brown toast with peanut butter or muesli and milk, a mix of protein and carbohydrates will keep you going and stop potential bingeing later on.

It is not an easy way to cut calories by missing a meal because when you skip a meal or go long periods without eating, you body will start to panic that it is not receiving food and will soon start to reserve food in the form of fat, just incase it happens again. This is what we call starvation mode and it makes you put on weight because fat is being stored unnecessarily. The same goes for when your go on a diet, lose weight, come off the diet and put it on again. This vicious cycle of losing and gaining weight will only make it harder for you each time because your body is reserving fat incase it is needed for when you don't eat enough. The best option is to eat enough throughout the day in order to not feel hungry. The way to do this is to eat plenty but not just anything, fill up on healthy nutritious foods that are low in calories (check out the good food list for ideas).

When advising people about what to eat I have often found them to be shocked at just how much food can be consumed in a healthy diet. When compared, it is possible to eat a mountain of healthy food for the same amount of calories and fat in a small take-away and feel ten times more satisfied and fuller for longer. So, again, fill up on the good stuff!

Another excellent way of filling-up to avoid hunger later on, is to choose a diet high in protein and soups. It has been proven that when compared to a diet high in carbohydrates or fat, a diet high in protein will keep you feeling fuller for much longer meaning that you are much less likely to dive for the snacks. A good guide to protein size should be around a quarter of your meal. Soup is also high on the list of filling options The mixture of liquid and food mixed together to create soup will make the stomach expand to feel full and remain that way for longer than drinking water before or after a meal. By drinking water before a meal it may curb hunger and result in consuming less food, however, this is not as effective as the mixture of food and liquid (soup) together. When consumed separately, liquids will expand the stomach but pass through, followed by solid food. Soup works in a magical way by expanding the stomach and remaining that way for much longer, thus making you feel fuller for longer. So, as well as being tasty and nutritious (as long as you choose the right kind!) it can also be a great meal choice.

11. Know your portion size

One of the easiest and most obvious ways of losing weight is to cut portion size. In fact it is so easy you probably won't even notice the change. A very common reason for gaining weight and being over-weight is as plain and simple as eating too much. The best way to cut down on portion size is to use plates and bowls that are smaller and drinking glasses that are tall and slim. It sounds silly but works for two reasons. The first is that you physically can't put too much food on your plate, and secondly, psychologically speaking, if you see a full plate your eyes send messages to your brain that your eating enough, while a big plate that is half empty screams diet. Moreover the habit of 'clearing the plate' can have serious consequences when it is a full large plate. We may not consciously realise we do it but filling and clearing our plates comes naturally to us, not a great habit if the plate is the size of a dustbin lid!

The same thing goes for when you choose less than saintly groceries or meals at a restaurant, always try to downsize. For example, if you love chocolate and choose this as your treat buy mini sized chocolate bars instead. The temptation to eat a full size bar will be gone but you can still enjoy your favourite treat. This theory can be applied to just about everything, ice creams can be found in smaller sized portions, sandwiches can be purchased that are not huge and most restaurants and cafes will be able to make smaller portions of a meal or drink on request. Another way in which you can cut portion size is to share when possible. Say you are in a cafe and your favourite slice of cake only comes in 'giant size' but you just can't pass it by, ask your friend to share it with you. It may seem obvious but if previously you would have eaten a slice by yourself, simply by sharing it, you have cut half the calories.

The stomach is roughly the size of a grapefruit, not very big when compared to the size of a regular dinner and well worth remembering when choosing the right portion size. Often we over-consume without noticing because we think about filling our plates or getting value for money with a 'meal deal' rather than what we actually need to fill our stomachs. Over time, portion sizes have increased so much that a take-away cola from a fast food joint that would have been considered large 15 years ago would today, in most places, be considered small. Food companies are trying to get us to consume more through value for money offers that seem like a bargain at the time but will not help our waistlines because a high percentage of foods that are on offer are unhealthy. So be aware of the right portion size and don't be tempted to consume more.

This is such an easy and subtle change that you probably won't even notice the difference and certainly in time you will find that the portion size you were originally used to is just too much. Your stomach is small but it has the capacity to expand to meet intake levels. If you regularly consume large portions of food your stomach will accommodate and tolerate these large portions. Likewise with smaller portions, after a couple of months of eating a healthy portion size you will find that you feel fuller, quicker and on a lot less food than before as your stomach will not be accustomed to eating large quantities of food. After this it will be easier to maintain portion size as long as you listen to your body for when you feel full and stop eating. While you don't want to feel hungry, it is also an unpleasant feeling to be over-full, nobody enjoys feeling nauseous and bloated. Over-eating will not only lead to instant unpleasant side effects but long term this extra food that is unnecessary for your body will be stored as fat unless it is burnt off by physical activity.

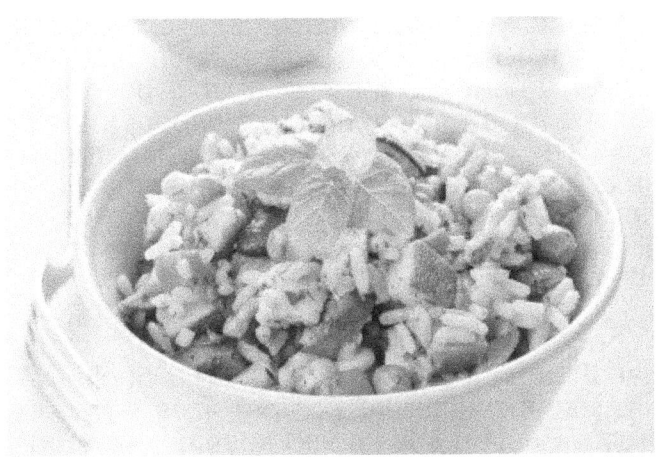

You can learn to gauge the right portion size for you by recognising the sensation of feeling full and therefore avoid over eating, then you will be able to lose and control your weight. If you are unsure about how hungry or full you feel, try imagining a scale of 1-10, where 1 means you are truly starving and your body is unable to function and 10 meaning you are so full you couldn't eat another bite. Think about how your body feels and honestly gauge where you are on the scale, it's time to eat when you are about a level 3; getting hungry but not starving and stop eating when you feel to be about a level 7. This is especially helpful during meals as a quick check can help you understand if you should stop eating.

Another way to check that you have the right portion size is to load half of your plate with vegetables, salad or fruit. A quarter of the plate is for protein (lean meat and fish should roughly be about the size of your palm or a deck of cards, and for a portion of cheese about the size of a matchbox). The last quarter is for complex carbohydrates and a small amount should be goods fats, maybe a small drizzle of olive oil. With this as a rough guide you are more likely to see how much of each food group you should be putting on your plate.

It has become especially difficult for women to understand the right portion size as, on a whole, we have gradually lost the different portion sizes between men and women. Restaurants serve the same size portion for both sexes and many of us tend to forget that a woman's body requires less calories than men. On average, men require 2500 calories and women 2000 a day, so for ladies a slightly smaller portion size is advisable to keep within the necessary daily calorie intake. Remember when cooking; a portion size for a female should be slightly smaller than that of a male, a daily difference of 500 calories, which roughly equates to a whole meal.

If you want to lose weight it is vital that you are not influenced by those around you. Don't feel pressurised into having bigger portions or unnecessary food by family, friends or even society. Some people find it helpful to tell those that they regularly eat and socialise with about their intentions to change their eating habits, so that they can understand and support. Others prefer not to voice the changes that they are making to their diets and see it more as subtle life changes. Neither way is right or wrong, think about which approach would be most helpful to you and to the alterations you are making to your diet and lifestyle. It greatly depends on the attitudes of your family and friends and if you think it would be helpful. Most of us have at least one person close to us that likes to dish out third portions and won't let you leave their house until you are stuffed with their food and carrying away six boxes of extras in case you are hungry later. You may even have someone that gets upset or offended if you don't eat all that they offer. Think carefully about the type of people you surround yourself with and instead of avoiding them or offending them you may find the best option is to clearly explain that your eating habits have changed and how important it is for you. Together you can make changes and compromises when you are in each other's company and food is involved.

Portion size plays an important role in not only losing weight but maintaining weight. In order to lose weight the body must be in a calorie deficit, normally by 250 to 1000 calories a day, through exercise and eating well, which will result in a healthy and steady weight loss of 0.5-2 lbs (maximum 1kg) a week. While many people are aware of this and can successfully lose weight there are many more people that find it difficult to maintain the weight loss. In order to do this. It's necessary to take an honest look at how much exercise and activity you do on a regular basis and therefore how many calories are needed to maintain this level. By keeping a close eye on these two factors when you have reached your target weight and you are gradually getting a feel of how much is enough you will be able to maintain it. It will take a few months and a sharp eye to keep track of triggers and pitfalls but eventually you will find a natural balance. Plus, once you have implemented all of these small changes and altered your habits it will be easier to see this as a regular way of life.

Eating healthy food you may assume allows you to eat as much as you want, While you can eat a much greater quantity of healthy low-fat food than you would high-fat calorie dense food, it still doesn't give you license to eat an endless limit. While it would be almost impossible to gain weight on a diet of only salad leaves other healthy foods can still be calorie dense and should be eaten in moderation if the aim is to lose weight. These include nuts and seeds, avocado, bananas and hummus which are all very healthy foods that contain an excellent array of vitamins, nutrients and healthy fats and are great to include in your diet, but are high in calories and are easily over consumed. It is possible to over-eat on a healthy diet, and as a result not lose weight, and in some cases it's even possible to gain weight. Before you start throwing out the healthy food and order a cheeseburger all you need to do is be aware of those foods that are high in calories, know how much is a good portion size and to limit yourself to that amount. If you know that stopping at just a small handful of nuts will be as likely as winning the lottery then find something else. Information is the key here, knowing what you are eating and having just a rough idea of it's calorie content, even if it's a healthy food, will help you make the right choices.

12. Eat for the right reasons

Primarily, the human body needs food to provide energy for it to function and for the activities you make your body do. If we eat for the wrong reasons and don't burn off the extra calories we gain weight. A perfect example of this is eating for emotional reasons. More and more people are turning to food for comfort when they face emotional disturbances. Nearly everyone has done this at some point and it's very common with both men and women. Ben and Jerry's ice cream may make you feel better for half an hour or so but the emotions will still be there, plus you probably now feel rather guilty and nauseous!

Another classic reason for eating when it is not necessary is 'because it was there'. Recognise and realise that this is not an adequate reason for consuming food. It may also help by not having unhealthy foods and drink in the house. If this is unavoidable then try not to have them in view. Display a tasty looking bowl of fruit and you will be more likely to choose this better option. Boredom, stress, anger, sadness, tiredness and pretty much every other emotion are all triggers for eating. To avoid the situation where these triggers ruin your new healthy lifestyle recognise when you are likely to raid the cupboard for food for the wrong reasons.

One perfect example of emotional eating was a client who had changed his eating habits and diet drastically. He had lost a lot of weight and was seeing great changes due to a new exercise program. He expressed how great he was feeling and was really enjoying his new lifestyle. One day he came to me and said that he had just had a big argument with his girlfriend and wanted to eat a huge hamburger and fries. This direct link of emotional upset and unhealthy eating nearly had him digressing. Once he realised what he was doing he was shocked at how he misused food. He didn't even realise what he was doing.

Food is not a support so the first step is recognising if you have any reasons for using food in a similar way. Stop and ask yourself for what reason do you want to eat. If it is an emotional one break the link and do something else. Again, use the hunger scale to judge your need to eat. Recognise what your personal triggers are and you will be able to avoid the pit-fall of overeating or eating badly when it occurs. If this is something that you suspect you do try writing down on your food diary if you were really hungry, and if not what was the reason for eating. You have to be totally honest with yourself, it can be very revealing and extremely helpful in understanding your motivations and triggers for eating.

The perfect alternative to eating is exercise. It releases feel good endorphins and de-stresses. You may not feel like it at the time but afterwards you will feel much better having had a quick jog in the fresh air rather than having eaten a baby elephant's weight in doughnuts. Another example of eating when unnecessary is at celebrations and restaurants. Never eat 'because it's there' or you feel peer pressure to do so, if you are full then stop. Be in control of what you eat and don't let anyone else tell you otherwise. It is not rude to refuse the fifth round of the buffet, it is logical. Don't eat food that you don't really like either, supermarkets and restaurants are full of different varieties of food so there is no need to eat things that you don't really like. If your friend likes Chinese take-away but you are not crazy for it, don't feel you have to eat it, choose something else. Healthy choices are in abundance so choose wisely and enjoy your food.

13. Understand your bad habits and break them

Everyone has ways in which they are less than perfect when it comes to eating and exercise but if we realise what they are, it becomes easier to alter them. If you can't open a huge bar of chocolate without eating it all (however much you tell yourself that it will be different this time!) avoid the risk of eating the whole king-size bar by buying small snack-size bars and just having one. The temptation to have just 'one more square' will be gone. Mentally it is easier because you know that the portion you are allowing yourself to have is in the wrapper already prepared for you, rather than leaving it up to you and your self-control to stop.

Pay attention to your eating habits and note when you are at risk of your healthy eating ways going out of the window. Say, for example, that you always fall for the huge muffin every time that you take a coffee. Once you have noted your pitfall you can do something to change it, pack a bag of dried fruit and nuts in your bag to nibble on instead. Another classic example is skipping a meal and a couple of hours later having a major snack-attack because you are hungry.

Try writing down what you eat and when, include what you were doing and anything else that you may find helpful in identifying your sabotages! There are so many different ways in which it is easy to end up reaching for the wrong things or too much of it but after a week or two of checking your ways you will notice bad habits that are sabotaging the healthier habits. Take just half an hour to think and plan ways that you can avoid these pitfalls. One of the best ways to avoid succumbing to bad habits is to not keep unhealthy food in the house but stock up on fruit and healthy treats instead. If it's not there then you won't be able to ruin all those good hours spent in the gym. You won't need to spend time thinking about it and trying to resist it either. Much better to have an inviting basket of fresh fruit out on display rather than a cupboard full of chocolate and cakes. You will be much more likely to choose the better option.

Planning and having an idea of what to cook and eat is a powerful way of taking control of your diet. By knowing what you need to buy for the week, what your going to cook and when, it is possible to eliminate those last minute panic meals of frozen pizza and fries. Studies have shown that the more one leaves meal times up to a last minute decision the more likely those meals are to be higher in fat, sugar and calories. Only a couple of minutes is needed to plan meals just a couple of days in advance so that the stress of decision making is avoided and healthier choices are more likely to be made.

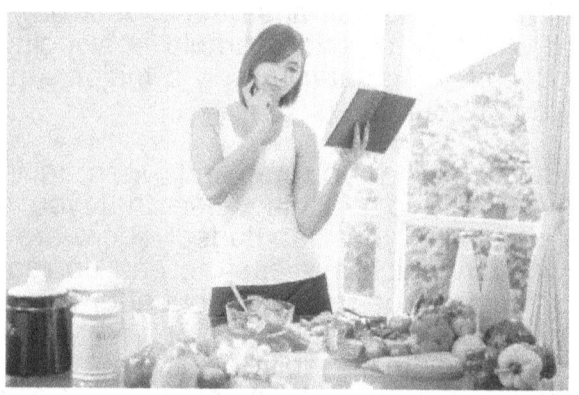

14. Speed up your metabolic rate

There are a few ways in which you can speed up your metabolic rate (how fast you burn calories), which in turn will mean that your body will burn more calories from day-to-day. One of the best ways to do this is to increase muscle mass as it means that someone with a high muscle mass, who consumes the same amount of calories as someone with a low muscle mass will burn many more calories, even during times of inactivity. This doesn't mean that you have to be built like the incredible hulk it just means that a little extra muscle requires more calories and in turn helps manage body weight.

Cardiovascular exercise is often considered the main type of exercise to perform for weight loss. It is great for burning calories and improving fitness but it is not the best way to increase muscle mass. By solely performing cardiovascular exercise you will miss out on the long term benefits of resistance training. Consider asking a professional fitness instructor to give you a basic resistance program alongside cardio training. This will also help tone areas of your body that you are not keen on. It is important that you do the exercises correctly so that you can avoid injury and to make sure that you are getting the maximum out of your sessions.

One thing to consider when increasing muscle mass is that your weight may increase too. This is common and more than likely doesn't mean that you are getting bigger or have increased fat percentage. Muscle weighs more than fat and therefore will increase the number on the scales even if your clothes feel looser and your belt is pulled in a notch tighter.

Don't pay to much attention to the numbers on the scale, in fact it can be very off putting to see that your weight is staying the same or even increasing. Some very slim and fit people, with a high muscle mass can weigh a considerable amount more than expected. Measuring your progress solely on the number on the scales can be very inaccurate. It is important that your body composition is made up of the right elements, which means a low body fat percentage and a good percentage of muscle mass, bone mass and also water; which will make up a significant percentage of body mass. The best way to measure progress is to get regularly weighed on body composition scales that have separate muscle mass and body fat readings. Most good gyms will be able to provide these and they can also be purchased. It is also not a good idea to weigh yourself too frequently since it takes time to change your body and lose weight. Once a week is more than enough to keep an eye on progress. Weighing yourself too often could lead to disappointment if you are not progressing like you thought you would.

Weight loss should not be rushed, as mentioned before, this is a change of lifestyle and eating habits, not a crash diet. The steadier the weight loss, the more chance there is that the weight will stay off for the long-run, so don't feel tempted to cut back drastically or lose more than the recommended amount. Instead of looking at the numbers, pay attention to how your clothes feel and how you feel in yourself. Has your energy increased? Can you run for longer and easier? Do you need to buy a new wardrobe?!

Also approach BMI (body mass index) measurements with caution as this takes into account only your height and weight, again, without muscle mass playing a part, meaning that very fit body builders or rugby players are considered morbidly obese. It can be an unreliable and inaccurate measurement of body composition. Not only can it mistakenly give the reading that some fit and muscle-bound bodies can be obese but it also works in reverse. Slim figures without muscle mass, that eat a very unhealthy diet can have a very healthy BMI which is reassuring for the individual but not an accurate representation. It doesn't necessarily mean that because they are slim and lean they are healthy. It could be the complete opposite and they have a very unhealthy diet and have incredibly poor fitness. If you are serious about being healthy and fit, it is best to visit a professional instructor who can advise on all areas of diet and fitness and will be able to accurately measure you and your progress.

Getting enough sleep is one of the most important elements of a healthy lifestyle. Not getting enough sleep or having irregular and sporadic sleep patterns can have a big knock-on effect to your metabolism. The body won't know when to store fat, when to shut down, or when to repair itself. Try sticking to a regular time for going to sleep and waking up and by getting at least 7-8 hours of sleep per night you will really be helping your metabolism.

The same principle goes for regular eating and as mentioned before not skipping meals. The more balanced and regular your eating habits are the more 'reassured' your body will be that it's going to get food and doesn't need to protect itself and go into starvation mode. This might seem dramatic but our bodies are just trying to do what's best to survive.

In recent years the small 6-8 meals a day concept has seen increased popularity and while studies have shown that eating regularly can help weight loss it can depend on your own lifestyle and personality to know if this concept will work for you. Obviously it takes more effort and judgement to prepare 6-8 meals of 250 calories everyday, and that's without taking into consideration when you are going to fit in the time to spread out the consumption of these meals in a busy working day. It has also been noted that this constant state of grazing can lead to over-eating because without strictly measuring the meals and controlling the portion sizes it can be easy to fall into a habit of constantly eating having blurred the lines of set meals. The benefit of eating every few hours is that your body doesn't have to digest big heavy meals and won't go long periods of time without food, an overall healthy balance. A more convenient and manageable way of getting these benefits and still maintaining a clear meal time schedule would be to stick to having three main meals a day (breakfast and lunch being the slightly bigger of those) but including small, healthy snacks in between to keep the energy levels up.

Another way to increase the metabolic rate is to drink green or oolong tea, as mentioned before, the benefits of green tea are many but green and oolong teas are also shown to rev-up the metabolism for a couple of hours due to the caffeine and catechin substances found in the teas. Research suggests that drinking two to four cups of either tea may push the body to burn 17% more calories than normal during moderately intense exercise for a short period of time. It has also been shown that certain foods can have a positive effect on boosting the metabolism including spicy foods as they contain chemical compounds that can kick the metabolism into a higher gear. However, the impact of foods and drinks on the metabolism is small compared to what you need for sustained weight loss. The best way to create an effective calorie burning body is to build muscle and stay active. The more you move during the day, the more calories you burn.

Everyone has a different metabolism that depends mainly on genetics and lifestyle. Ultimately it is up to you to find out the right portion size and the right types of food that your body needs. Some people find it difficult to put weight on whilst others find it extremely hard to lose and maintain a healthy weight, we are all different. By being aware of what and how much you are consuming it is possible to have a good idea of what it takes to control your weight. You can make changes to increase your metabolism to a certain point but also try to understand what and how much you need in your diet in order to lose, gain or maintain weight. Once you have found the right balance you will have more control over the results you can get from you body.

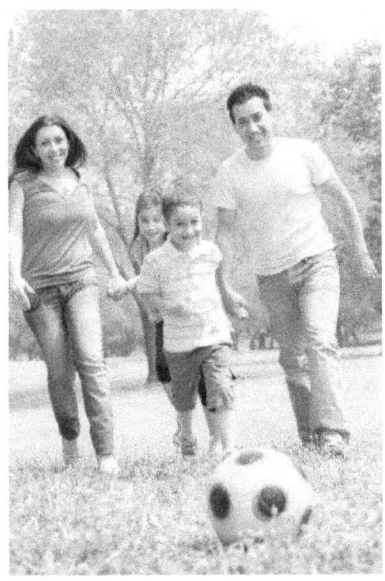

15. Understand your body genetics and accept them

While there are many things that we can change about our bodies and many ways that we can improve the way our bodies look there are also limits because of the pre-disposed genetics passed down from our parents. To understand what you can improve through diet and exercise take a look at old photos of what you consider to be you at your very best 'body wise'. Notice how your body looks and you will be able to understand what you can alter and what your limits are. However much you may hate a certain body part, if it is an area genetically formed this way, there is a limit to what you can do to change this naturally- exercising and dieting until you break will not help.

Even when you had your very 'best body' the chances are that there was at least one area that you wished you could change and these are the things that you must learn to accept as part of you. Depending on the shape of body we were blessed with, we will be pre-disposed to putting on weight in certain areas, again something you are likely to have in common with one of your parents. For some of us, when we put on weight the first place it will go to is the tummy area and even though it's not impossible it's unlikely that gaining a six-pack stomach will be possible however much sweat and hard work is carried out. Other people carry weight on their lower half and will find that it is harder to control these areas because in some ways it is like fighting genetics.

It's not all bad news and it shouldn't be an excuse to avoid exercise. Yes there are going to be areas you may never be 100% happy with but we can change and improve a lot through the right diet and the right exercise.

So accept that you may never have the lean, slim legs of the models in the magazines because both your parents have legs like tree trunks and seek professional advice for exercises that will help you improve what you do have. The aim is to know and love your body, treat it well and feed it a healthy, balanced diet that will reward you by feeling good on the inside and looking great on the outside.

The 'good food' list

The following is a list of foods you can choose from to include in your diet and a rough portion guide. Remember to use a small plate!!!

Carbohydrates:
Brown/ whole grain bread (1 piece/ slice)
Brown rice (1/4 plate size)
Pasta, ideally whole grain/ brown (1/4 plate size)
Noodles, good quality (1/4 plate size)
Oats, cous cous, orzo, barley or quinoa (1/4 plate size)
Sweet potato (1/4 plate size)
Boiled, plain mashed or jacket potato (1/4 plate size)
Crackers and rice cakes (4-5 medium sized)
Low in sugar and natural cereals, porridge oats, granola or muesli (small bowl)

Protein:
Fish (1 piece, size of closed fist)
Lean meats like chicken, turkey, occasionally beef or pork (about the size of a deck of cards)
Eggs cooked in a healthy way; omelet, scrambled, poached, boiled etc (equivalent 1-2)
Beans and pulses like chick peas and lentils (1/4 plate size)
Nuts and seeds (a small handful)
Low-fat cheese or cottage cheese (small amount, size of your thumb)
Low-fat milk (1 cup)
Low in sugar and fat, natural yogurt (1 small pot)
Hummus (tablespoon)

All types of fruit, vegetable and salads without condiments or marination. Small amounts of banana, avocado and dried fruit for weight loss purposes (approximately 1/2 plate).

Soups can also be included but homemade varieties are best since ready-made soups often contain high amounts of sugar, salt and fat.

Drinks:
Water (minimum 8 glasses a day)
Low-fat milk (to be included in protein section)
Teas without sugars and a little low-fat milk
Coffee without sugar and a little low-fat milk
Natural fruit juice (maximum 1 small glass a day)

Condiments, seasonings and extras:
All spices, peppers and herbs
Extra virgin olive oil
Home made tomato sauces and purees (those that don't contain extra salt and sugar etc)
Garlic
All types of seeds
Pesto
Natural honey (small amount)
Low-fat vinaigrette
Many others (check the nutritional information label for more details)

Treat:
One small treat every other day. For example, a small glass of wine, a few squares of chocolate, 2-3 biscuits. This can be increased to a small treat every day only if you are exercising vigorously everyday and eating appropriate amounts of healthy food for the rest of your daily consumption. However, some treats are worse than others, try to go for 'healthier' treats that contain something nutritious about them like dark chocolate that contains antioxidants, or flapjack that contains oats and raisons. Keep the calorie count of this treat to 200.

Example

Each meal that you have (breakfast, lunch and dinner) should contain a portion of good quality carbohydrates, protein and salad / vegetables / fruit. Snacks in between meals (and when necessary) should ideally be something nutritious like fruit, whole-grain crackers or a small handful of nuts and dried fruit.

An example of a day's plan of food for a average female would look something like this:

Breakfast:
Carbohydrates- one slice of brown toast
Protein- one boiled egg
Grilled tomatoes

Snack:
Banana

Lunch:
Carbohydrates- quarter of a small plate of brown rice
Protein- palm sized grilled chicken breast, cooked with herbs or spices
Half a plate of mixed salad with a little olive oil
Portion of mixed fruit

Snack:
Small handful of mixed unsalted nuts and dried apricots

Dinner:
Carbohydrates- quarter of a small plate of pasta
Protein- one medium sized piece of grilled salmon
Half a plate of boiled or steamed mixed vegetables

This is a basic example, it is up to you to be creative and choose from the 'good food' list for meals.

What is classed as a 'good food'?

It is important not to think of the 'good food' list as a divide between foods that are permitted and foods that are forbidden or 'bad'. The 'good food' list is more of a guideline for healthy foods which should make up the vast majority of your everyday eating. There are other 'good foods' that are not included on this list and you can tell if they are 'good foods' as they have a few simple criteria in common:

They haven't changed much from their natural and original state- a banana still resembles a banana on the tree, whereas a crisp doesn't look like a potato because it has been heavily processed.
'Good foods' don't last for months, they will go off if left as they don't contain lots of preservatives.
Generally they contain fewer than five or six ingredients.
'Good foods' don't need any artificial flavour or additives.
They don't contain ingredients that you can't pronounce, have numbers in them or that you don't recognise.
Sugar is not listed as their main ingredient or one of the first three ingredients.
They satisfy you and don't leave you feeling hungry shortly after eating them.
They don't make you feel gassy, uncomfortable or bloated.

The perfect multi-meal ingredient list

Pasta (ideally whole wheat)	Free range eggs	Broccoli
Sweet potato or regular potato	Tinned tuna	Carrots
Brown rice (or something similar like cous cous)	Mixed beans	Courgettes
Whole grain brown bread	Low-fat cheese	Tomatoes
	Free range skinless chicken breast	Spinach
	Skimmed or semi-skimmed milk	Onions

This list of 16 ingredients has been devised as a basic shopping list, suitable for all, from which you can create over 30 different meals. It comprises cheap, healthy and readily available ingredients that are highly versatile. If you were to purchase only the ingredients on this list you would easily have enough possibilities to feed even a fussy family for a minimum of two weeks. And while they may seem like 'normal' ingredients and you may already have at least a few of the ingredients in your kitchen it's the ideal stock list to make so many meals.

Each ingredient has been carefully chosen for not only it's versatility but for the nutritional qualities it contains. The list has been balanced in order to include a mixture of complex carbohydrates, quality protein and nutritious vegetables. The ingredients included hit the right balance between being highly nutritional foods while still being available in every supermarket and not being unusual in anyway. There are no 'scary' ingredients you don't know what to do with it! Also because each ingredient can be used in multiple dishes, with a little planning, there will be very minimal wastage. This is unlike those unusual, special ingredients you only purchase for one meal and then have to throw the remainder away because you don't know what else to use it with.

While a few store cupboard essentials are required in order to make meals with these ingredients they are basic things like cooking oil and herbs which you can find in every kitchen.

They might not be the most culinary spectacular ingredients but this list is for quick and simple, everyday lunches and dinners when you want healthy with no hassle. This is a 'no-excuse' ingredient list that takes the stress out of deciding what to purchase. It's 'no-excuse' because even if you have very limited knowledge on nutrition and your cooking skills peak at boiling water then you can make healthy, fresh meals without fuss. If is also ideal for anyone that has limited time to shop, prepare and cook meals because with only these ingredients it is possible to make an array of lunches and dinners all in a short space of time.

Of course this is a guide and if you have an allergy, intolerance or dislike to one or more of the ingredients you can simply exchange it for a similar type of ingredient. Likewise if you are a vegetarian or you have specific dietary needs. Meat can be exchanged for a different protein source like tofu or Quorn.

Whilst the ingredients are simple, you can jazz-up basic meals using spices and herbs. A dash of lemon can be used to flavour boiled courgettes or oregano can be sprinkled on tomatoes with a drizzle of extra virgin olive oil. With a little imagination you can use these simple ingredients to create incredible meals.

This list is designed for lunches and dinners and doesn't include breakfast foods or snacks. It is highly advised that a variety of fruit is purchased alongside this list to provide in-between meal snacks and to eat after meals too.

To increase the longevity of the vegetables it is a good idea to purchase a mixture of fresh and frozen so that you always have a supply on-hand. Likewise with the chicken, purchasing fresh chicken is ideal, however, freezing it is a great option if you don't intend to use it straight away.

Here are just a few meal suggestions:

-Crustless quiches; vegetable, potato, bean

-Soups; hearty bean, vegetable, potato, chicken and rice

-Omelettes; onion, potato, cheese, tomato, vegetable

-Pasta bakes; cheese, tuna, chicken, vegetables, bean

-Casseroles; beans, vegetables, pasta, chicken, potato, rice

-Sandwiches; tomato, cheese, egg, tuna, carrot and courgette strips

-Salads using tomato and grated carrot and courgette; tuna, pasta, potato, egg, chicken, bean, rice, crouton, cheese

-Stir-fry; vegetables, chicken, rice, bean

-Pasta; tuna, cooked with whisked egg, beans, tomatoes, vegetables

-Grilled, stuffed, chicken breast

-Fish cakes

-Plus, don't forget all the ways you can cook potatoes, eggs and chicken

Cost comparison of buying ingredients and cooking meals compared with buying ready meals and takeaways from the supermarket (UK prices 2014)

We have already established that it can be very beneficial for our waistlines to home-cook meals rather than eating out or getting take-aways but how about the difference in price? Here we compare the cost of stocking up on ingredients and cooking meals to buying ready-made.

Research is based on lunches and dinners for two people over two weeks (ie. 14 lunches and 14 dinners or 28 meals)

Buying a mix of branded and supermarket branded ingredients (taken from the perfect multi-meal ingredient list) for an average couple to make 28 different meals:
Pasta, 1kg penne 98p
Potatoes, 4 large baking 98p
Rice, 1kg brown £1.78
Bread, 4x 800g fresh whole meal loaf £4

Eggs, 15 pack free range £2
Tuna, 3x 160g tins £3
Beans, 3x 400g tinned mix £2.10
Cheese, 450g low-fat £2.74
Chicken breasts, 1kg free range £13.98
Milk, 2x 6 pints semi skimmed £2.96

Broccoli, 500g fresh 69p
Carrots, 1kg fresh 75p
Courgettes, 1kg fresh £1.50
Tomatoes, 2x 6 pack fresh £1.38
Spinach, 350g fresh £1.50
Onions, 500kg 35p

Total £40.69
Average cost per meal for two people £1.45

The supermarket takeaway and ready meal option:
The very cheapest supermarket ready meal costs £1 for one person, as does a pre-made supermarket sandwich. Two weeks worth for two people would cost £56.
Average supermarket ready meal for two people costs £3.50. Two weeks worth would cost £98.
A simple supermarket Chinese takeaway including rice, chicken korma and onion bhajis costs £4.85. Two weeks worth would cost £135.80.

Average total cost of a mixture of the above meal options £96.60
Average cost per meal, of these three options, for two people £3.45

So the average price of a meal when cooked from brought ingredients is £1.45 and the average price for a ready made meal is £3.45. That's well over double the price for each meal!

A little bit about the author

Well I am a globe-trotting, exercise fanatic, fruit-eating machine that loves tea and gelato, but not together. Although I did find a recipe for milky-tea flavoured gelato, I am yet to try it and feel it could either be a disaster or possible the world's greatest find!

I have found the world of nutrition fascinating ever since training at a professional dance school in England. I learnt, from a young age how nutrition can change the way our bodies feel and have a dramatic effect on health and well-being. This continues to be my personal reason for aiming for a healthy, balanced diet. Even as a dancer, I had never wanted to be super skinny. I craved that healthy, fit body that comes only from treating it well. Long hours spent dancing, day after day, were punishing to my body and energy. I found it imperative to look after myself from the inside in order to let my body do what I was asking of it without getting ill or injured. Through trial and error (ie. don't drink too much the night before an important class) I learnt a lot and even though I have not physically asked so much of my body since it is something that I have continued to live by; a way of maintaining a healthy weight and healthy body but being able to enjoy good food without feeling deprived.

I moved on from dancing and entered the fitness industry where professional training and qualifications helped my understanding and truly fired my interest in providing information and knowledge to clients that were wanting to feel and look better. I learnt just how important it is for the body to be active and that when exercise is used in the right way it can help control weight and change the body shape. While healthy eating is the key to weight management, activity and exercise work alongside a good diet to help make weight management much easier. More than a weight controlling tool it can also be just a bit fun! Throughout my time in the fitness industry I have taught all sorts of types of exercise from aqua combat to yoga and most things in between. I found that the best thing about teaching those classes was seeing the participants leaving class a little pink-faced having had a good workout but ultimately smiling and happy. Those exercise endorphins really make you feel great!

From here I was fortunate to have the chance to work on cruise ships and see a bit of the world. After the initial excitement of constantly having a huge array or amazing foods available and certainly over indulging for probably a bit too long, I realised my body didn't feel good and instead I took advantage of all the foods that were better for me. Through personal experience I was proving that not only can a bad diet affect the body physically by putting on weight, feeling bloated and many other symptoms it also has a powerful link to how you feel such as increasing irritability, lowering concentration and creating mood swings to name just a few.

Through travelling it was interesting to witness different culture's relationship with food and dieting. Some think eating just one big meal a day is best others believe not eating after 6 is important and in some cultures starting the day with something sweet seems to be the way. By experiencing the different ways in which nutrition is looked upon I hope I have picked up the best points of many different attitudes and made sense of them. My husband's family is Italian and having a traditional Italian mother-in-law, who cooks-up an incredible cuisine has really opened my eyes. As a nation Italy has a relatively low percentage of the population who are obese and yet Italians are obsessed with food and eating. If thinking and talking about food was to relate to the actual number of obese people, well nearly every Italian would be obese but they are not! While spending many years being immersed in this new culture I learnt a great deal about the Italian nation's eating habits and the reasons behind their healthy lifestyle. Many of these elements have been incorporated into this guide.

I went on to qualify as a nutrition and weight management consultant to further my knowledge and help advise clients. It was this qualification and many years of studying exercise, healthy living and nutrition that lead me to want to come up with a way of taking all the information we regularly get bombarded with be it via the media, friendly advice, professional advice or the latest dieting trends and try to make sense out of it all. My aim was to find a straight forward way of getting back to a simple, natural way of eating that would be maintainable over a lifetime. Through friends, relatives and colleagues, I have witnessed the effects of just about every diet going with very mixed results. What strikes me most about all diets is just how hard it is to maintain them for longer than... maybe a week. It also became shockingly apparent how dieting is such a constant feature of so many peoples lives. It seems that even in this day and age we haven't managed to come up with a truly effective and healthy way of managing body weight. Also the restrictions that so many diets impose means that dieters are missing out on vital food groups and therefore nutrients. This means that they may lose weight in the short term but won't be genuinely healthy. This seemed ludicrous to me and the complete opposite of what a diet should be: aiming for optimum health.

It was my intention to not overload readers with nutritional detail and information but to deliver the key elements in easy to understand, relevant and realistic key points. Countless diet books have been written all promising amazing things and often offering long explanations to the complicated and expensive ways in which to achieve the wonder of weight loss. These books will tell you what you can and can't eat and when to eat it. Well I personally feel my soul leaving my body just thinking about this joyless routine! My aim was to tell the truth- weight management doesn't have to be complicated or punishing it just involves identifying what could be better and changing a few things about the current diet for healthier options. Our lifestyles are influenced by so many elements; the people around us, how we were brought up and modern culture just to name a few. Sometimes we need to be strong to identify any negative influences and alter them so we can benefit long-term. This leads to a key concept of making healthy changes; to embrace the new lifestyle and don't hold on to bad habits that pull you back into unhealthy living.

I hope that by following this golden guide it can lead you to dietary health for life.

For more information, personal nutrition consultation and the latest news about fitness and nutrition please visit:
revfitnessandnutrition.wordpress.com